Diabetes Record

I0428578

Date	AM Glucose	Food/Liquid
		Breakfast
Meds	**PM Glucose**	Lunch
		Dinner
		Exercise

Date	AM Glucose	Food/Liquid
		Breakfast
Meds	**PM Glucose**	Lunch
		Dinner
		Exercise

Date	AM Glucose	Food/Liquid
		Breakfast
Meds	**PM Glucose**	Lunch
		Dinner
		Exercise

Date	AM Glucose	Food/Liquid
		Breakfast
Meds	**PM Glucose**	Lunch
		Dinner
		Exercise

Diabetes Record

Date	AM Glucose	Food/Liquid
		Breakfast
Meds	PM Glucose	Lunch
		Dinner
		Exercise

Date	AM Glucose	Food/Liquid
		Breakfast
Meds	PM Glucose	Lunch
		Dinner
		Exercise

Date	AM Glucose	Food/Liquid
		Breakfast
Meds	PM Glucose	Lunch
		Dinner
		Exercise

Date	AM Glucose	Food/Liquid
		Breakfast
Meds	PM Glucose	Lunch
		Dinner
		Exercise

Diabetes Record

Date	AM Glucose	Food/Liquid
		Breakfast
Meds	PM Glucose	Lunch
		Dinner
		Exercise
Date	AM Glucose	Food/Liquid
		Breakfast
Meds	PM Glucose	Lunch
		Dinner
		Exercise
Date	AM Glucose	Food/Liquid
		Breakfast
Meds	PM Glucose	Lunch
		Dinner
		Exercise
Date	AM Glucose	Food/Liquid
		Breakfast
Meds	PM Glucose	Lunch
		Dinner
		Exercise

Diabetes Record

Date	AM Glucose	Food/Liquid		
		Breakfast		
Meds	PM Glucose	Lunch		
		Dinner		
		Exercise		

Date	AM Glucose	Food/Liquid		
		Breakfast		
Meds	PM Glucose	Lunch		
		Dinner		
		Exercise		

Date	AM Glucose	Food/Liquid		
		Breakfast		
Meds	PM Glucose	Lunch		
		Dinner		
		Exercise		

Date	AM Glucose	Food/Liquid		
		Breakfast		
Meds	PM Glucose	Lunch		
		Dinner		
		Exercise		

Diabetes Record

Date	AM Glucose	Food/Liquid
		Breakfast
		Lunch
Meds	PM Glucose	Dinner
		Exercise
Date	AM Glucose	Food/Liquid
		Breakfast
		Lunch
Meds	PM Glucose	Dinner
		Exercise
Date	AM Glucose	Food/Liquid
		Breakfast
		Lunch
Meds	PM Glucose	Dinner
		Exercise
Date	AM Glucose	Food/Liquid
		Breakfast
		Lunch
Meds	PM Glucose	Dinner
		Exercise

Diabetes Record

Date	AM Glucose	Food/Liquid
		Breakfast
Meds	PM Glucose	Lunch
		Dinner
		Exercise
Date	AM Glucose	Food/Liquid
		Breakfast
Meds	PM Glucose	Lunch
		Dinner
		Exercise
Date	AM Glucose	Food/Liquid
		Breakfast
Meds	PM Glucose	Lunch
		Dinner
		Exercise
Date	AM Glucose	Food/Liquid
		Breakfast
Meds	PM Glucose	Lunch
		Dinner
		Exercise

Diabetes Record

Date	AM Glucose	Food/Liquid
		Breakfast
		Lunch
Meds	PM Glucose	Dinner
		Exercise

Date	AM Glucose	Food/Liquid
		Breakfast
		Lunch
Meds	PM Glucose	Dinner
		Exercise

Date	AM Glucose	Food/Liquid
		Breakfast
		Lunch
Meds	PM Glucose	Dinner
		Exercise

Date	AM Glucose	Food/Liquid
		Breakfast
		Lunch
Meds	PM Glucose	Dinner
		Exercise

Diabetes Record

Date	AM Glucose	Food/Liquid
		Breakfast
		Lunch
Meds	PM Glucose	Dinner
		Exercise

Date	AM Glucose	Food/Liquid
		Breakfast
		Lunch
Meds	PM Glucose	Dinner
		Exercise

Date	AM Glucose	Food/Liquid
		Breakfast
		Lunch
Meds	PM Glucose	Dinner
		Exercise

Date	AM Glucose	Food/Liquid
		Breakfast
		Lunch
Meds	PM Glucose	Dinner
		Exercise

Diabetes Record

Date	AM Glucose	Food/Liquid
		Breakfast
		Lunch
Meds	PM Glucose	Dinner
		Exercise

Date	AM Glucose	Food/Liquid
		Breakfast
		Lunch
Meds	PM Glucose	Dinner
		Exercise

Date	AM Glucose	Food/Liquid
		Breakfast
		Lunch
Meds	PM Glucose	Dinner
		Exercise

Date	AM Glucose	Food/Liquid
		Breakfast
		Lunch
Meds	PM Glucose	Dinner
		Exercise

Diabetes Record

Date	AM Glucose	Food/Liquid
		Breakfast
		Lunch
Meds	PM Glucose	Dinner
		Exercise

Date	AM Glucose	Food/Liquid
		Breakfast
		Lunch
Meds	PM Glucose	Dinner
		Exercise

Date	AM Glucose	Food/Liquid
		Breakfast
		Lunch
Meds	PM Glucose	Dinner
		Exercise

Date	AM Glucose	Food/Liquid
		Breakfast
		Lunch
Meds	PM Glucose	Dinner
		Exercise

Diabetes Record

Date	AM Glucose	Food/Liquid
		Breakfast
Meds	PM Glucose	Lunch
		Dinner
		Exercise
Date	AM Glucose	Food/Liquid
		Breakfast
Meds	PM Glucose	Lunch
		Dinner
		Exercise
Date	AM Glucose	Food/Liquid
		Breakfast
Meds	PM Glucose	Lunch
		Dinner
		Exercise
Date	AM Glucose	Food/Liquid
		Breakfast
Meds	PM Glucose	Lunch
		Dinner
		Exercise

Diabetes Record

Date	AM Glucose	Food/Liquid	
		Breakfast	
Meds	PM Glucose	Lunch	
		Dinner	
		Exercise	
Date	AM Glucose	Food/Liquid	
		Breakfast	
Meds	PM Glucose	Lunch	
		Dinner	
		Exercise	
Date	AM Glucose	Food/Liquid	
		Breakfast	
Meds	PM Glucose	Lunch	
		Dinner	
		Exercise	
Date	AM Glucose	Food/Liquid	
		Breakfast	
Meds	PM Glucose	Lunch	
		Dinner	
		Exercise	

Diabetes Record

Date	AM Glucose	Food/Liquid
		Breakfast
		Lunch
Meds	PM Glucose	Dinner
		Exercise

Date	AM Glucose	Food/Liquid
		Breakfast
		Lunch
Meds	PM Glucose	Dinner
		Exercise

Date	AM Glucose	Food/Liquid
		Breakfast
		Lunch
Meds	PM Glucose	Dinner
		Exercise

Date	AM Glucose	Food/Liquid
		Breakfast
		Lunch
Meds	PM Glucose	Dinner
		Exercise

Diabetes Record

Date	AM Glucose	Food/Liquid
		Breakfast
		Lunch
Meds	PM Glucose	Dinner
		Exercise
Date	AM Glucose	Food/Liquid
		Breakfast
		Lunch
Meds	PM Glucose	Dinner
		Exercise
Date	AM Glucose	Food/Liquid
		Breakfast
		Lunch
Meds	PM Glucose	Dinner
		Exercise
Date	AM Glucose	Food/Liquid
		Breakfast
		Lunch
Meds	PM Glucose	Dinner
		Exercise

Diabetes Record

Date	AM Glucose	Food/Liquid		
		Breakfast		
Meds	PM Glucose	Lunch		
		Dinner		
		Exercise		
Date	AM Glucose	Food/Liquid		
		Breakfast		
Meds	PM Glucose	Lunch		
		Dinner		
		Exercise		
Date	AM Glucose	Food/Liquid		
		Breakfast		
Meds	PM Glucose	Lunch		
		Dinner		
		Exercise		
Date	AM Glucose	Food/Liquid		
		Breakfast		
Meds	PM Glucose	Lunch		
		Dinner		
		Exercise		

Diabetes Record

Date	AM Glucose	Food/Liquid
		Breakfast
		Lunch
Meds	PM Glucose	Dinner
		Exercise

Date	AM Glucose	Food/Liquid
		Breakfast
		Lunch
Meds	PM Glucose	Dinner
		Exercise

Date	AM Glucose	Food/Liquid
		Breakfast
		Lunch
Meds	PM Glucose	Dinner
		Exercise

Date	AM Glucose	Food/Liquid
		Breakfast
		Lunch
Meds	PM Glucose	Dinner
		Exercise

Diabetes Record

Date	AM Glucose	Food/Liquid
		Breakfast
		Lunch
Meds	PM Glucose	Dinner
		Exercise

Date	AM Glucose	Food/Liquid
		Breakfast
		Lunch
Meds	PM Glucose	Dinner
		Exercise

Date	AM Glucose	Food/Liquid
		Breakfast
		Lunch
Meds	PM Glucose	Dinner
		Exercise

Date	AM Glucose	Food/Liquid
		Breakfast
		Lunch
Meds	PM Glucose	Dinner
		Exercise

Diabetes Record

Date	AM Glucose	Food/Liquid		
		Breakfast		
		Lunch		
Meds	PM Glucose	Dinner		
		Exercise		
Date	AM Glucose	Food/Liquid		
		Breakfast		
		Lunch		
Meds	PM Glucose	Dinner		
		Exercise		
Date	AM Glucose	Food/Liquid		
		Breakfast		
		Lunch		
Meds	PM Glucose	Dinner		
		Exercise		
Date	AM Glucose	Food/Liquid		
		Breakfast		
		Lunch		
Meds	PM Glucose	Dinner		
		Exercise		

Diabetes Record

Date	AM Glucose	Food/Liquid
		Breakfast
Meds	**PM Glucose**	**Lunch**
		Dinner
		Exercise
Date	**AM Glucose**	**Food/Liquid**
		Breakfast
Meds	**PM Glucose**	**Lunch**
		Dinner
		Exercise
Date	**AM Glucose**	**Food/Liquid**
		Breakfast
Meds	**PM Glucose**	**Lunch**
		Dinner
		Exercise
Date	**AM Glucose**	**Food/Liquid**
		Breakfast
Meds	**PM Glucose**	**Lunch**
		Dinner
		Exercise

Diabetes Record

Date	AM Glucose	Food/Liquid
		Breakfast
		Lunch
Meds	PM Glucose	Dinner
		Exercise

Date	AM Glucose	Food/Liquid
		Breakfast
		Lunch
Meds	PM Glucose	Dinner
		Exercise

Date	AM Glucose	Food/Liquid
		Breakfast
		Lunch
Meds	PM Glucose	Dinner
		Exercise

Date	AM Glucose	Food/Liquid
		Breakfast
		Lunch
Meds	PM Glucose	Dinner
		Exercise

Diabetes Record

Date	AM Glucose	Food/Liquid		
		Breakfast		
Meds	PM Glucose	Lunch		
		Dinner		
		Exercise		

Date	AM Glucose	Food/Liquid		
		Breakfast		
Meds	PM Glucose	Lunch		
		Dinner		
		Exercise		

Date	AM Glucose	Food/Liquid		
		Breakfast		
Meds	PM Glucose	Lunch		
		Dinner		
		Exercise		

Date	AM Glucose	Food/Liquid		
		Breakfast		
Meds	PM Glucose	Lunch		
		Dinner		
		Exercise		

Diabetes Record

Date	AM Glucose	Food/Liquid
		Breakfast
Meds	PM Glucose	Lunch
		Dinner
		Exercise
Date	AM Glucose	Food/Liquid
		Breakfast
Meds	PM Glucose	Lunch
		Dinner
		Exercise
Date	AM Glucose	Food/Liquid
		Breakfast
Meds	PM Glucose	Lunch
		Dinner
		Exercise
Date	AM Glucose	Food/Liquid
		Breakfast
Meds	PM Glucose	Lunch
		Dinner
		Exercise

Date	AM Glucose	Food/Liquid
		Breakfast
Meds	PM Glucose	Lunch
		Dinner
		Exercise

Date	AM Glucose	Food/Liquid
		Breakfast
Meds	PM Glucose	Lunch
		Dinner
		Exercise

Date	AM Glucose	Food/Liquid
		Breakfast
Meds	PM Glucose	Lunch
		Dinner
		Exercise

Date	AM Glucose	Food/Liquid
		Breakfast
Meds	PM Glucose	Lunch
		Dinner
		Exercise

Diabetes Record

Date	AM Glucose	Food/Liquid		
		Breakfast		
Meds	PM Glucose	Lunch		
		Dinner		
		Exercise		
Date	AM Glucose	Food/Liquid		
		Breakfast		
Meds	PM Glucose	Lunch		
		Dinner		
		Exercise		
Date	AM Glucose	Food/Liquid		
		Breakfast		
Meds	PM Glucose	Lunch		
		Dinner		
		Exercise		
Date	AM Glucose	Food/Liquid		
		Breakfast		
Meds	PM Glucose	Lunch		
		Dinner		
		Exercise		

Diabetes Record

Date	AM Glucose	Food/Liquid		
		Breakfast		
Meds	PM Glucose	Lunch		
		Dinner		
		Exercise		
Date	AM Glucose	Food/Liquid		
		Breakfast		
Meds	PM Glucose	Lunch		
		Dinner		
		Exercise		
Date	AM Glucose	Food/Liquid		
		Breakfast		
Meds	PM Glucose	Lunch		
		Dinner		
		Exercise		
Date	AM Glucose	Food/Liquid		
		Breakfast		
Meds	PM Glucose	Lunch		
		Dinner		
		Exercise		

Diabetes Record

Date	AM Glucose	Food/Liquid
		Breakfast
		Lunch
Meds	PM Glucose	Dinner
		Exercise
Date	AM Glucose	Food/Liquid
		Breakfast
		Lunch
Meds	PM Glucose	Dinner
		Exercise
Date	AM Glucose	Food/Liquid
		Breakfast
		Lunch
Meds	PM Glucose	Dinner
		Exercise
Date	AM Glucose	Food/Liquid
		Breakfast
		Lunch
Meds	PM Glucose	Dinner
		Exercise

Diabetes Record

Date	AM Glucose	Food/Liquid
		Breakfast
		Lunch
Meds	PM Glucose	Dinner
		Exercise

Date	AM Glucose	Food/Liquid
		Breakfast
		Lunch
Meds	PM Glucose	Dinner
		Exercise

Date	AM Glucose	Food/Liquid
		Breakfast
		Lunch
Meds	PM Glucose	Dinner
		Exercise

Date	AM Glucose	Food/Liquid
		Breakfast
		Lunch
Meds	PM Glucose	Dinner
		Exercise

Diabetes Record

Date	AM Glucose	Food/Liquid		
		Breakfast		
Meds	PM Glucose	Lunch		
		Dinner		
		Exercise		
Date	AM Glucose	Food/Liquid		
		Breakfast		
Meds	PM Glucose	Lunch		
		Dinner		
		Exercise		
Date	AM Glucose	Food/Liquid		
		Breakfast		
Meds	PM Glucose	Lunch		
		Dinner		
		Exercise		
Date	AM Glucose	Food/Liquid		
		Breakfast		
Meds	PM Glucose	Lunch		
		Dinner		
		Exercise		

Diabetes Record

Date	AM Glucose	Food/Liquid
		Breakfast
		Lunch
Meds	PM Glucose	Dinner
		Exercise
Date	AM Glucose	Food/Liquid
		Breakfast
		Lunch
Meds	PM Glucose	Dinner
		Exercise
Date	AM Glucose	Food/Liquid
		Breakfast
		Lunch
Meds	PM Glucose	Dinner
		Exercise
Date	AM Glucose	Food/Liquid
		Breakfast
		Lunch
Meds	PM Glucose	Dinner
		Exercise

Diabetes Record

Date	AM Glucose	Food/Liquid		
		Breakfast		
		Lunch		
Meds	PM Glucose	Dinner		
		Exercise		
Date	AM Glucose	Food/Liquid		
		Breakfast		
		Lunch		
Meds	PM Glucose	Dinner		
		Exercise		
Date	AM Glucose	Food/Liquid		
		Breakfast		
		Lunch		
Meds	PM Glucose	Dinner		
		Exercise		
Date	AM Glucose	Food/Liquid		
		Breakfast		
		Lunch		
Meds	PM Glucose	Dinner		
		Exercise		

Date	AM Glucose	Food/Liquid
		Breakfast
		Lunch
Meds	PM Glucose	Dinner
		Exercise
Date	AM Glucose	Food/Liquid
		Breakfast
		Lunch
Meds	PM Glucose	Dinner
		Exercise
Date	AM Glucose	Food/Liquid
		Breakfast
		Lunch
Meds	PM Glucose	Dinner
		Exercise
Date	AM Glucose	Food/Liquid
		Breakfast
		Lunch
Meds	PM Glucose	Dinner
		Exercise

Diabetes Record

Date	AM Glucose	Food/Liquid
		Breakfast
Meds	PM Glucose	Lunch
		Dinner
		Exercise
Date	AM Glucose	Food/Liquid
		Breakfast
Meds	PM Glucose	Lunch
		Dinner
		Exercise
Date	AM Glucose	Food/Liquid
		Breakfast
Meds	PM Glucose	Lunch
		Dinner
		Exercise
Date	AM Glucose	Food/Liquid
		Breakfast
Meds	PM Glucose	Lunch
		Dinner
		Exercise

Diabetes Record

Date	AM Glucose	Food/Liquid	
		Breakfast	
Meds	PM Glucose	Lunch	
		Dinner	
		Exercise	
Date	AM Glucose	Food/Liquid	
		Breakfast	
Meds	PM Glucose	Lunch	
		Dinner	
		Exercise	
Date	AM Glucose	Food/Liquid	
		Breakfast	
Meds	PM Glucose	Lunch	
		Dinner	
		Exercise	
Date	AM Glucose	Food/Liquid	
		Breakfast	
Meds	PM Glucose	Lunch	
		Dinner	
		Exercise	

Diabetes Record

Date	AM Glucose	Food/Liquid
		Breakfast
		Lunch
Meds	PM Glucose	Dinner
		Exercise

Date	AM Glucose	Food/Liquid
		Breakfast
		Lunch
Meds	PM Glucose	Dinner
		Exercise

Date	AM Glucose	Food/Liquid
		Breakfast
		Lunch
Meds	PM Glucose	Dinner
		Exercise

Date	AM Glucose	Food/Liquid
		Breakfast
		Lunch
Meds	PM Glucose	Dinner
		Exercise

Diabetes Record

Date	AM Glucose	Food/Liquid	
		Breakfast	
		Lunch	
Meds	**PM Glucose**	**Dinner**	
		Exercise	
Date	**AM Glucose**	**Food/Liquid**	
		Breakfast	
		Lunch	
Meds	**PM Glucose**	**Dinner**	
		Exercise	
Date	**AM Glucose**	**Food/Liquid**	
		Breakfast	
		Lunch	
Meds	**PM Glucose**	**Dinner**	
		Exercise	
Date	**AM Glucose**	**Food/Liquid**	
		Breakfast	
		Lunch	
Meds	**PM Glucose**	**Dinner**	
		Exercise	

Date	AM Glucose	Food/Liquid
		Breakfast
		Lunch
Meds	PM Glucose	Dinner
		Exercise

Date	AM Glucose	Food/Liquid
		Breakfast
		Lunch
Meds	PM Glucose	Dinner
		Exercise

Date	AM Glucose	Food/Liquid
		Breakfast
		Lunch
Meds	PM Glucose	Dinner
		Exercise

Date	AM Glucose	Food/Liquid
		Breakfast
		Lunch
Meds	PM Glucose	Dinner
		Exercise

Diabetes Record

Date	AM Glucose	Food/Liquid
		Breakfast
		Lunch
Meds	PM Glucose	Dinner
		Exercise

Date	AM Glucose	Food/Liquid
		Breakfast
		Lunch
Meds	PM Glucose	Dinner
		Exercise

Date	AM Glucose	Food/Liquid
		Breakfast
		Lunch
Meds	PM Glucose	Dinner
		Exercise

Date	AM Glucose	Food/Liquid
		Breakfast
		Lunch
Meds	PM Glucose	Dinner
		Exercise

Date	AM Glucose	Food/Liquid
		Breakfast
Meds	PM Glucose	Lunch
		Dinner
		Exercise
Date	AM Glucose	Food/Liquid
		Breakfast
Meds	PM Glucose	Lunch
		Dinner
		Exercise
Date	AM Glucose	Food/Liquid
		Breakfast
Meds	PM Glucose	Lunch
		Dinner
		Exercise
Date	AM Glucose	Food/Liquid
		Breakfast
Meds	PM Glucose	Lunch
		Dinner
		Exercise

Date	AM Glucose	Food/Liquid
		Breakfast
		Lunch
Meds	PM Glucose	Dinner
		Exercise

Date	AM Glucose	Food/Liquid
		Breakfast
		Lunch
Meds	PM Glucose	Dinner
		Exercise

Date	AM Glucose	Food/Liquid
		Breakfast
		Lunch
Meds	PM Glucose	Dinner
		Exercise

Date	AM Glucose	Food/Liquid
		Breakfast
		Lunch
Meds	PM Glucose	Dinner
		Exercise

Diabetes Record

Date	AM Glucose	Food/Liquid
		Breakfast
		Lunch
Meds	PM Glucose	Dinner
		Exercise

Date	AM Glucose	Food/Liquid
		Breakfast
		Lunch
Meds	PM Glucose	Dinner
		Exercise

Date	AM Glucose	Food/Liquid
		Breakfast
		Lunch
Meds	PM Glucose	Dinner
		Exercise

Date	AM Glucose	Food/Liquid
		Breakfast
		Lunch
Meds	PM Glucose	Dinner
		Exercise

Diabetes Record

Date	AM Glucose	Food/Liquid
		Breakfast
Meds	**PM Glucose**	Lunch
		Dinner
		Exercise

Date	AM Glucose	Food/Liquid
		Breakfast
Meds	**PM Glucose**	Lunch
		Dinner
		Exercise

Date	AM Glucose	Food/Liquid
		Breakfast
Meds	**PM Glucose**	Lunch
		Dinner
		Exercise

Date	AM Glucose	Food/Liquid
		Breakfast
Meds	**PM Glucose**	Lunch
		Dinner
		Exercise

Date	AM Glucose	Food/Liquid
		Breakfast
Meds	PM Glucose	Lunch
		Dinner
		Exercise
Date	AM Glucose	Food/Liquid
		Breakfast
Meds	PM Glucose	Lunch
		Dinner
		Exercise
Date	AM Glucose	Food/Liquid
		Breakfast
Meds	PM Glucose	Lunch
		Dinner
		Exercise
Date	AM Glucose	Food/Liquid
		Breakfast
Meds	PM Glucose	Lunch
		Dinner
		Exercise

Diabetes Record

Date	AM Glucose	Food/Liquid		
		Breakfast		
Meds	PM Glucose	Lunch		
		Dinner		
		Exercise		
Date	AM Glucose	Food/Liquid		
		Breakfast		
Meds	PM Glucose	Lunch		
		Dinner		
		Exercise		
Date	AM Glucose	Food/Liquid		
		Breakfast		
Meds	PM Glucose	Lunch		
		Dinner		
		Exercise		
Date	AM Glucose	Food/Liquid		
		Breakfast		
Meds	PM Glucose	Lunch		
		Dinner		
		Exercise		

Diabetes Record

Date	AM Glucose	Food/Liquid
		Breakfast
Meds	PM Glucose	Lunch
		Dinner
		Exercise
Date	AM Glucose	Food/Liquid
		Breakfast
Meds	PM Glucose	Lunch
		Dinner
		Exercise
Date	AM Glucose	Food/Liquid
		Breakfast
Meds	PM Glucose	Lunch
		Dinner
		Exercise
Date	AM Glucose	Food/Liquid
		Breakfast
Meds	PM Glucose	Lunch
		Dinner
		Exercise

Diabetes Record

Date	AM Glucose	Food/Liquid
		Breakfast
Meds	PM Glucose	Lunch
		Dinner
		Exercise

Date	AM Glucose	Food/Liquid
		Breakfast
Meds	PM Glucose	Lunch
		Dinner
		Exercise

Date	AM Glucose	Food/Liquid
		Breakfast
Meds	PM Glucose	Lunch
		Dinner
		Exercise

Date	AM Glucose	Food/Liquid
		Breakfast
Meds	PM Glucose	Lunch
		Dinner
		Exercise

Date	AM Glucose	Food/Liquid		
		Breakfast		
Meds	PM Glucose	Lunch		
		Dinner		
		Exercise		
Date	AM Glucose	Food/Liquid		
		Breakfast		
Meds	PM Glucose	Lunch		
		Dinner		
		Exercise		
Date	AM Glucose	Food/Liquid		
		Breakfast		
Meds	PM Glucose	Lunch		
		Dinner		
		Exercise		
Date	AM Glucose	Food/Liquid		
		Breakfast		
Meds	PM Glucose	Lunch		
		Dinner		
		Exercise		

Diabetes Record

Date	AM Glucose	Food/Liquid
		Breakfast
Meds	PM Glucose	Lunch
		Dinner
		Exercise
Date	AM Glucose	Food/Liquid
		Breakfast
Meds	PM Glucose	Lunch
		Dinner
		Exercise
Date	AM Glucose	Food/Liquid
		Breakfast
Meds	PM Glucose	Lunch
		Dinner
		Exercise
Date	AM Glucose	Food/Liquid
		Breakfast
Meds	PM Glucose	Lunch
		Dinner
		Exercise

Date	AM Glucose	Food/Liquid
		Breakfast
Meds	PM Glucose	Lunch
		Dinner
		Exercise
Date	AM Glucose	Food/Liquid
		Breakfast
Meds	PM Glucose	Lunch
		Dinner
		Exercise
Date	AM Glucose	Food/Liquid
		Breakfast
Meds	PM Glucose	Lunch
		Dinner
		Exercise
Date	AM Glucose	Food/Liquid
		Breakfast
Meds	PM Glucose	Lunch
		Dinner
		Exercise

Diabetes Record

Date	AM Glucose	Food/Liquid
		Breakfast
		Lunch
Meds	PM Glucose	Dinner
		Exercise

Date	AM Glucose	Food/Liquid
		Breakfast
		Lunch
Meds	PM Glucose	Dinner
		Exercise

Date	AM Glucose	Food/Liquid
		Breakfast
		Lunch
Meds	PM Glucose	Dinner
		Exercise

Date	AM Glucose	Food/Liquid
		Breakfast
		Lunch
Meds	PM Glucose	Dinner
		Exercise

Diabetes Record

Date	AM Glucose	Food/Liquid
		Breakfast
		Lunch
Meds	PM Glucose	Dinner
		Exercise
Date	AM Glucose	Food/Liquid
		Breakfast
		Lunch
Meds	PM Glucose	Dinner
		Exercise
Date	AM Glucose	Food/Liquid
		Breakfast
		Lunch
Meds	PM Glucose	Dinner
		Exercise
Date	AM Glucose	Food/Liquid
		Breakfast
		Lunch
Meds	PM Glucose	Dinner
		Exercise

Date	AM Glucose	Food/Liquid
		Breakfast
		Lunch
Meds	PM Glucose	Dinner
		Exercise

Date	AM Glucose	Food/Liquid
		Breakfast
		Lunch
Meds	PM Glucose	Dinner
		Exercise

Date	AM Glucose	Food/Liquid
		Breakfast
		Lunch
Meds	PM Glucose	Dinner
		Exercise

Date	AM Glucose	Food/Liquid
		Breakfast
		Lunch
Meds	PM Glucose	Dinner
		Exercise

Date	AM Glucose	Food/Liquid
		Breakfast
Meds	**PM Glucose**	**Lunch**
		Dinner
		Exercise
Date	AM Glucose	Food/Liquid
		Breakfast
Meds	**PM Glucose**	**Lunch**
		Dinner
		Exercise
Date	AM Glucose	Food/Liquid
		Breakfast
Meds	**PM Glucose**	**Lunch**
		Dinner
		Exercise
Date	AM Glucose	Food/Liquid
		Breakfast
Meds	**PM Glucose**	**Lunch**
		Dinner
		Exercise

Diabetes Record

Date	AM Glucose	Food/Liquid		
		Breakfast		
Meds	PM Glucose	Lunch		
		Dinner		
		Exercise		

Date	AM Glucose	Food/Liquid		
		Breakfast		
Meds	PM Glucose	Lunch		
		Dinner		
		Exercise		

Date	AM Glucose	Food/Liquid		
		Breakfast		
Meds	PM Glucose	Lunch		
		Dinner		
		Exercise		

Date	AM Glucose	Food/Liquid		
		Breakfast		
Meds	PM Glucose	Lunch		
		Dinner		
		Exercise		

Diabetes Record

Date	AM Glucose	Food/Liquid
		Breakfast
		Lunch
Meds	PM Glucose	Dinner
		Exercise
Date	AM Glucose	Food/Liquid
		Breakfast
		Lunch
Meds	PM Glucose	Dinner
		Exercise
Date	AM Glucose	Food/Liquid
		Breakfast
		Lunch
Meds	PM Glucose	Dinner
		Exercise
Date	AM Glucose	Food/Liquid
		Breakfast
		Lunch
Meds	PM Glucose	Dinner
		Exercise

Date	AM Glucose	Food/Liquid
		Breakfast
		Lunch
Meds	PM Glucose	Dinner
		Exercise
Date	AM Glucose	Food/Liquid
		Breakfast
		Lunch
Meds	PM Glucose	Dinner
		Exercise
Date	AM Glucose	Food/Liquid
		Breakfast
		Lunch
Meds	PM Glucose	Dinner
		Exercise
Date	AM Glucose	Food/Liquid
		Breakfast
		Lunch
Meds	PM Glucose	Dinner
		Exercise

Diabetes Record

Date	AM Glucose	Food/Liquid
		Breakfast
Meds	PM Glucose	Lunch
		Dinner
		Exercise
Date	AM Glucose	Food/Liquid
		Breakfast
Meds	PM Glucose	Lunch
		Dinner
		Exercise
Date	AM Glucose	Food/Liquid
		Breakfast
Meds	PM Glucose	Lunch
		Dinner
		Exercise
Date	AM Glucose	Food/Liquid
		Breakfast
Meds	PM Glucose	Lunch
		Dinner
		Exercise

Diabetes Record

Date	AM Glucose	Food/Liquid
		Breakfast
		Lunch
Meds	PM Glucose	Dinner
		Exercise
Date	AM Glucose	Food/Liquid
		Breakfast
		Lunch
Meds	PM Glucose	Dinner
		Exercise
Date	AM Glucose	Food/Liquid
		Breakfast
		Lunch
Meds	PM Glucose	Dinner
		Exercise
Date	AM Glucose	Food/Liquid
		Breakfast
		Lunch
Meds	PM Glucose	Dinner
		Exercise

Date	AM Glucose	Food/Liquid
		Breakfast
		Lunch
Meds	PM Glucose	Dinner
		Exercise
Date	AM Glucose	Food/Liquid
		Breakfast
		Lunch
Meds	PM Glucose	Dinner
		Exercise
Date	AM Glucose	Food/Liquid
		Breakfast
		Lunch
Meds	PM Glucose	Dinner
		Exercise
Date	AM Glucose	Food/Liquid
		Breakfast
		Lunch
Meds	PM Glucose	Dinner
		Exercise

Diabetes Record

Date	AM Glucose	Food/Liquid
		Breakfast
Meds	PM Glucose	Lunch
		Dinner
		Exercise
Date	AM Glucose	Food/Liquid
		Breakfast
Meds	PM Glucose	Lunch
		Dinner
		Exercise
Date	AM Glucose	Food/Liquid
		Breakfast
Meds	PM Glucose	Lunch
		Dinner
		Exercise
Date	AM Glucose	Food/Liquid
		Breakfast
Meds	PM Glucose	Lunch
		Dinner
		Exercise

Diabetes Record

Date	AM Glucose	Food/Liquid
		Breakfast
		Lunch
Meds	PM Glucose	Dinner
		Exercise

Date	AM Glucose	Food/Liquid
		Breakfast
		Lunch
Meds	PM Glucose	Dinner
		Exercise

Date	AM Glucose	Food/Liquid
		Breakfast
		Lunch
Meds	PM Glucose	Dinner
		Exercise

Date	AM Glucose	Food/Liquid
		Breakfast
		Lunch
Meds	PM Glucose	Dinner
		Exercise

Date	AM Glucose	Food/Liquid		
		Breakfast		
Meds	PM Glucose	Lunch		
		Dinner		
		Exercise		

Date	AM Glucose	Food/Liquid		
		Breakfast		
Meds	PM Glucose	Lunch		
		Dinner		
		Exercise		

Date	AM Glucose	Food/Liquid		
		Breakfast		
Meds	PM Glucose	Lunch		
		Dinner		
		Exercise		

Date	AM Glucose	Food/Liquid		
		Breakfast		
Meds	PM Glucose	Lunch		
		Dinner		
		Exercise		

Diabetes Record

Date	AM Glucose	Food/Liquid
		Breakfast
		Lunch
Meds	PM Glucose	Dinner
		Exercise

Date	AM Glucose	Food/Liquid
		Breakfast
		Lunch
Meds	PM Glucose	Dinner
		Exercise

Date	AM Glucose	Food/Liquid
		Breakfast
		Lunch
Meds	PM Glucose	Dinner
		Exercise

Date	AM Glucose	Food/Liquid
		Breakfast
		Lunch
Meds	PM Glucose	Dinner
		Exercise

Diabetes Record

Date	AM Glucose	Food/Liquid
		Breakfast
		Lunch
Meds	PM Glucose	Dinner
		Exercise

Date	AM Glucose	Food/Liquid
		Breakfast
		Lunch
Meds	PM Glucose	Dinner
		Exercise

Date	AM Glucose	Food/Liquid
		Breakfast
		Lunch
Meds	PM Glucose	Dinner
		Exercise

Date	AM Glucose	Food/Liquid
		Breakfast
		Lunch
Meds	PM Glucose	Dinner
		Exercise

Diabetes Record

Date	AM Glucose	Food/Liquid
		Breakfast
		Lunch
Meds	PM Glucose	Dinner
		Exercise

Date	AM Glucose	Food/Liquid
		Breakfast
		Lunch
Meds	PM Glucose	Dinner
		Exercise

Date	AM Glucose	Food/Liquid
		Breakfast
		Lunch
Meds	PM Glucose	Dinner
		Exercise

Date	AM Glucose	Food/Liquid
		Breakfast
		Lunch
Meds	PM Glucose	Dinner
		Exercise

Date	AM Glucose	Food/Liquid
		Breakfast
Meds	PM Glucose	Lunch
		Dinner
		Exercise

Date	AM Glucose	Food/Liquid
		Breakfast
Meds	PM Glucose	Lunch
		Dinner
		Exercise

Date	AM Glucose	Food/Liquid
		Breakfast
Meds	PM Glucose	Lunch
		Dinner
		Exercise

Date	AM Glucose	Food/Liquid
		Breakfast
Meds	PM Glucose	Lunch
		Dinner
		Exercise

Diabetes Record

Date	AM Glucose	Food/Liquid
		Breakfast
Meds	PM Glucose	Lunch
		Dinner
		Exercise

Date	AM Glucose	Food/Liquid
		Breakfast
Meds	PM Glucose	Lunch
		Dinner
		Exercise

Date	AM Glucose	Food/Liquid
		Breakfast
Meds	PM Glucose	Lunch
		Dinner
		Exercise

Date	AM Glucose	Food/Liquid
		Breakfast
Meds	PM Glucose	Lunch
		Dinner
		Exercise

Diabetes Record

Date	AM Glucose	Food/Liquid
		Breakfast
Meds	PM Glucose	Lunch
		Dinner
		Exercise
Date	AM Glucose	Food/Liquid
		Breakfast
Meds	PM Glucose	Lunch
		Dinner
		Exercise
Date	AM Glucose	Food/Liquid
		Breakfast
Meds	PM Glucose	Lunch
		Dinner
		Exercise
Date	AM Glucose	Food/Liquid
		Breakfast
Meds	PM Glucose	Lunch
		Dinner
		Exercise

Date	AM Glucose	Food/Liquid
		Breakfast
Meds	PM Glucose	Lunch
		Dinner
		Exercise
Date	AM Glucose	Food/Liquid
		Breakfast
Meds	PM Glucose	Lunch
		Dinner
		Exercise
Date	AM Glucose	Food/Liquid
		Breakfast
Meds	PM Glucose	Lunch
		Dinner
		Exercise
Date	AM Glucose	Food/Liquid
		Breakfast
Meds	PM Glucose	Lunch
		Dinner
		Exercise

Diabetes Record

Date	AM Glucose	Food/Liquid		
		Breakfast		
		Lunch		
Meds	PM Glucose	Dinner		
		Exercise		
Date	AM Glucose	Food/Liquid		
		Breakfast		
		Lunch		
Meds	PM Glucose	Dinner		
		Exercise		
Date	AM Glucose	Food/Liquid		
		Breakfast		
		Lunch		
Meds	PM Glucose	Dinner		
		Exercise		
Date	AM Glucose	Food/Liquid		
		Breakfast		
		Lunch		
Meds	PM Glucose	Dinner		
		Exercise		

Diabetes Record

Date	AM Glucose	Food/Liquid
		Breakfast
Meds	PM Glucose	Lunch
		Dinner
		Exercise
Date	AM Glucose	Food/Liquid
		Breakfast
Meds	PM Glucose	Lunch
		Dinner
		Exercise
Date	AM Glucose	Food/Liquid
		Breakfast
Meds	PM Glucose	Lunch
		Dinner
		Exercise
Date	AM Glucose	Food/Liquid
		Breakfast
Meds	PM Glucose	Lunch
		Dinner
		Exercise

Diabetes Record

Date	AM Glucose	Food/Liquid	
		Breakfast	
		Lunch	
Meds	PM Glucose	Dinner	
		Exercise	
Date	AM Glucose	Food/Liquid	
		Breakfast	
		Lunch	
Meds	PM Glucose	Dinner	
		Exercise	
Date	AM Glucose	Food/Liquid	
		Breakfast	
		Lunch	
Meds	PM Glucose	Dinner	
		Exercise	
Date	AM Glucose	Food/Liquid	
		Breakfast	
		Lunch	
Meds	PM Glucose	Dinner	
		Exercise	